Jacob's Journey

Living with Type 1 Diabetes

By Deanna Kleiman
Illustrated by Kirsten Brieger

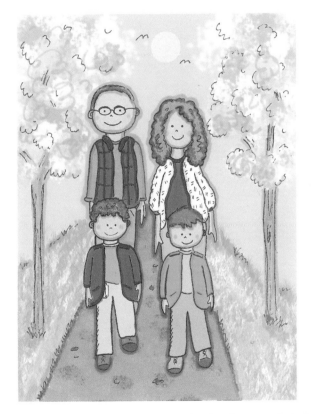

Dedicated with all my love, to Jacob, the bravest boy I know.

And to David, the best, most supportive brother I know.

*With special thanks to my loving husband Ira,
without whom I could never have done this.*

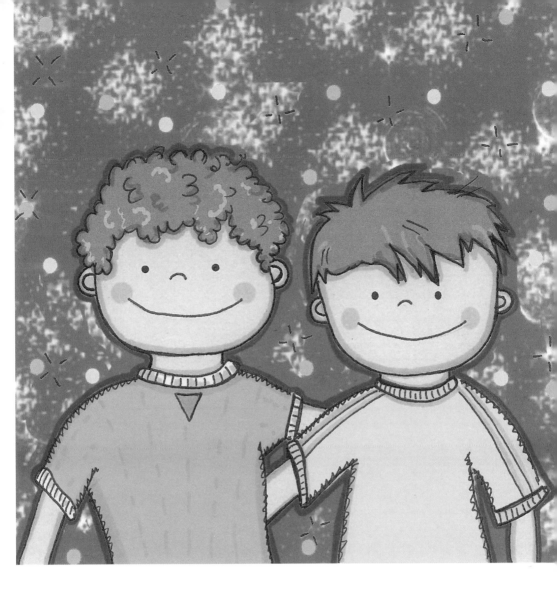

Hi, my name is Jacob and I am 8 years old.

I have a twin brother named David
and he is 8 too.

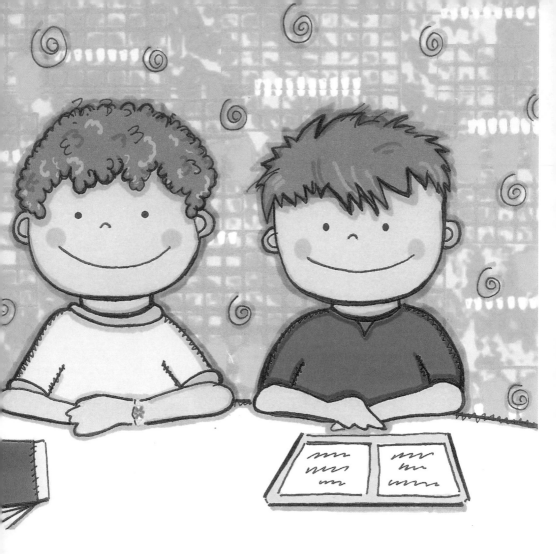

We are alike in some ways, but we have
a lot of differences too.

Like I have diabetes and David doesn't.

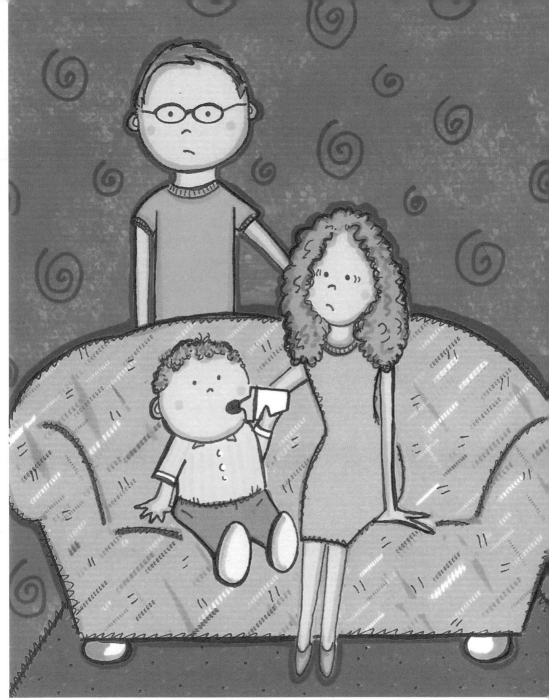

My parents noticed something was wrong when I was 2 years old.

I was thirsty all the time and drinking a lot! I was also wetting the bed a lot, and sometimes I hardly had any energy at all.

3

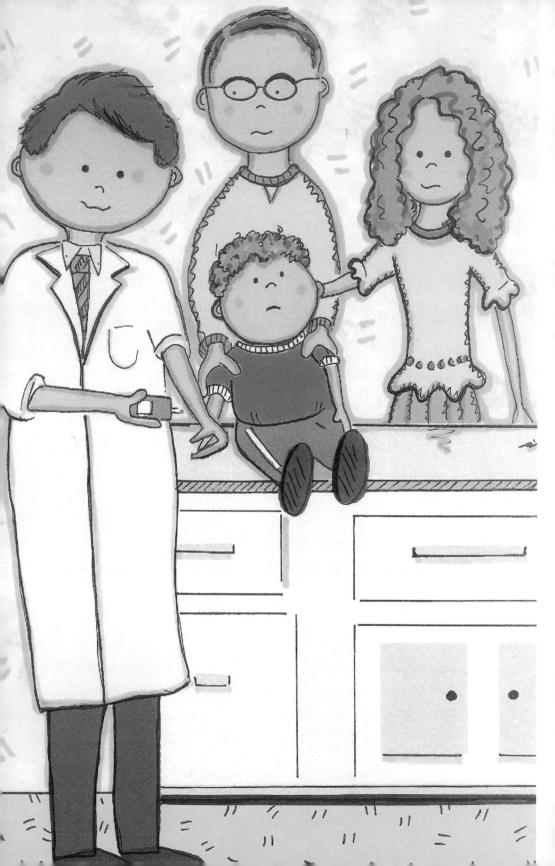

So my mom and dad took me to the doctor and he did a test that shows how much sugar is in your blood stream.

Well that test showed that the amount of sugar in my blood was very, very high and that meant I had something called "Type 1 Diabetes". This means that an organ in your body called your pancreas is not working properly, and is not producing something called "insulin". Insulin is what keeps too much sugar from getting into your blood.

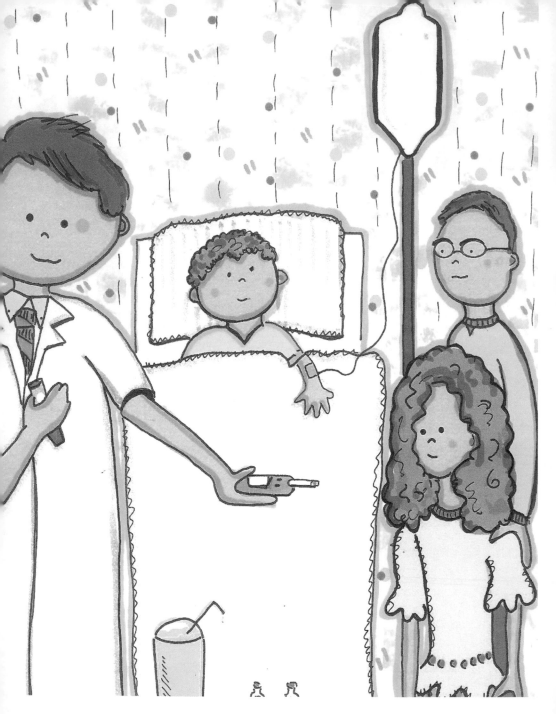

So we had to go to the hospital right from the doctor's office.

We stayed in the hospital for 3 days, so the doctors there could give me insulin to make sure there wasn't too much sugar in my blood.

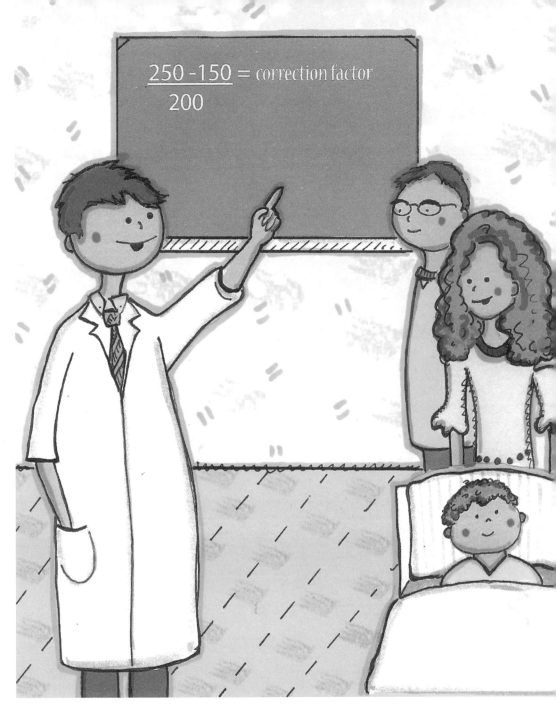

$$\frac{250 - 150}{200} = \text{correction factor}$$

They also taught my parents how to poke my finger to test my blood sugar, and what "glucose level" is right for me. Glucose level is just a fancy way of saying how much sugar is in your blood.

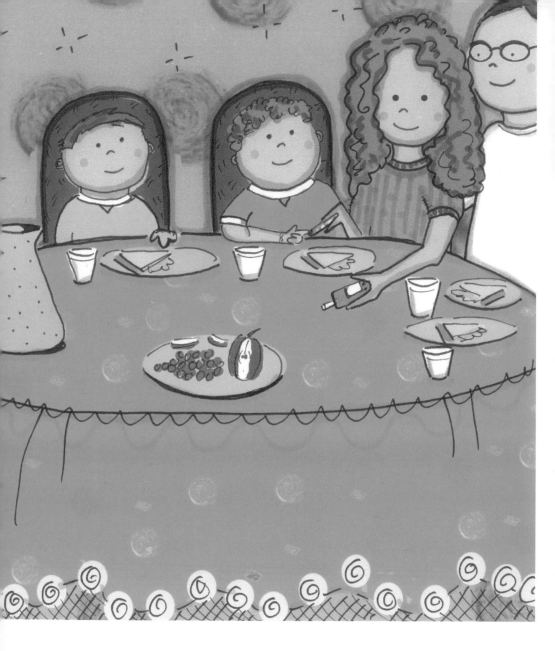

At first I cried every time someone poked my finger to test my blood. I was only 2 years old. But then I got used to it and pretty soon it didn't hurt at all.

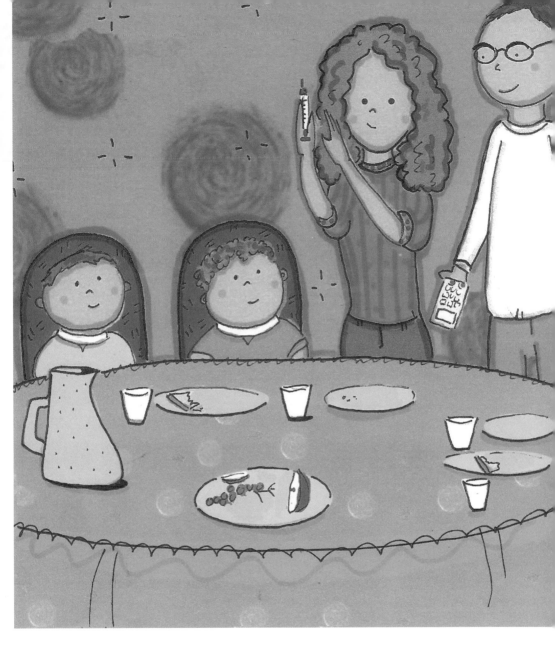

The doctors in the hospital also told my parents that they would have to give me a shot full of insulin every time I ate or drank anything. Then the doctors showed them how to figure out how much insulin to give me so they would know how to do it themselves.

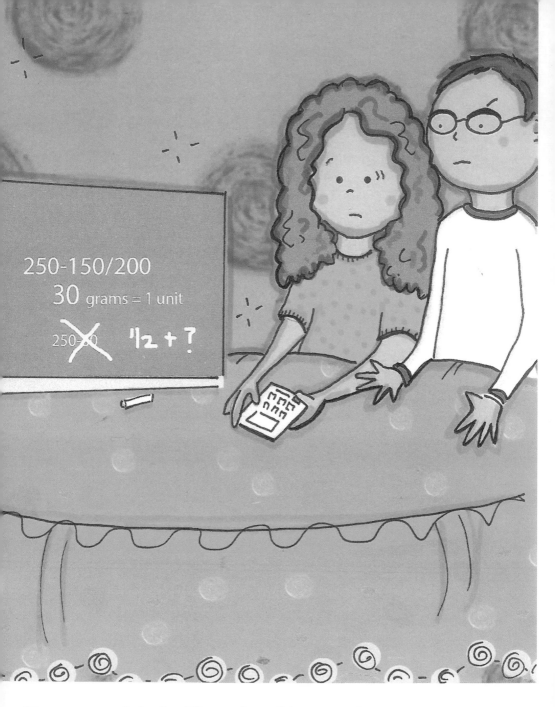

My mom and dad told me that this scared them very much. They weren't doctors so they had never given anyone a shot before, and they were afraid they might not figure out the amount of insulin correctly.

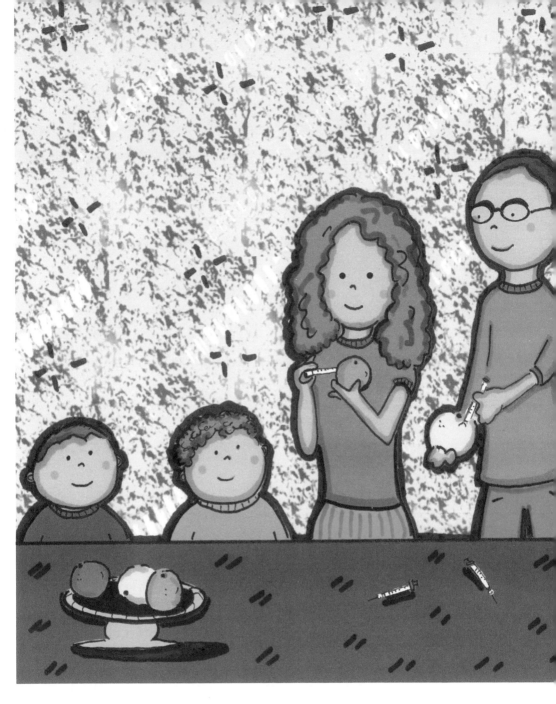

But the doctors and nurses at the hospital showed my
parents how to do it, and they even practiced giving shots
on oranges and grapefruits so they would feel comfortable
giving them to me!

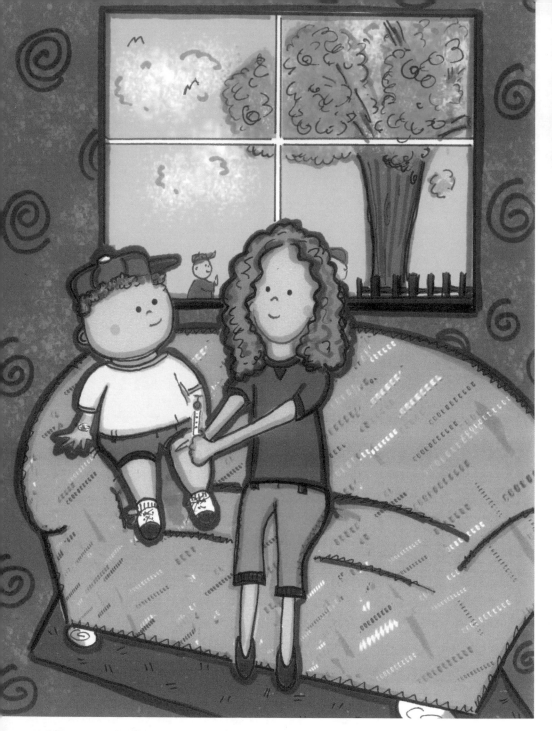

At first I cried every single time I had to have a shot, but pretty soon, just like when I had to have my finger poked, I didn't even feel the shots anymore!

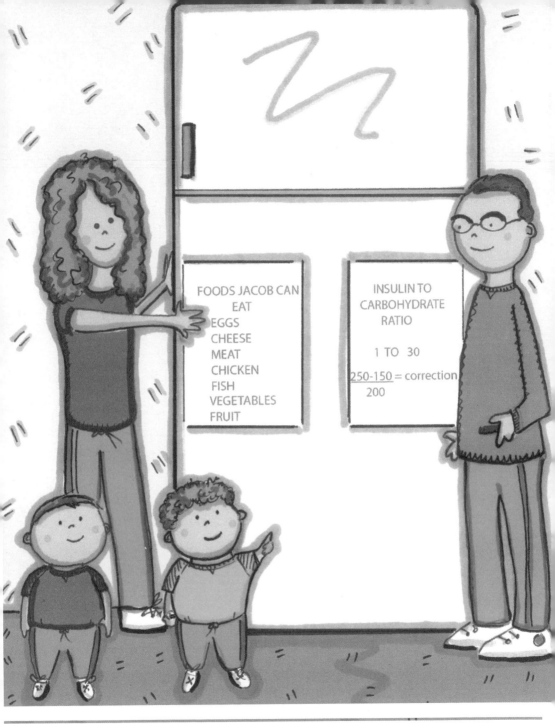

FOODS JACOB CAN
EAT
EGGS
CHEESE
MEAT
CHICKEN
FISH
VEGETABLES
FRUIT

INSULIN TO
CARBOHYDRATE
RATIO

1 TO 30

250-150 = correction
200

When we got home from the hospital my mom and dad put special charts up on the refrigerator. These charts showed what kinds of food I was allowed to eat, and the special formula they had to use to figure out how much insulin to give me.

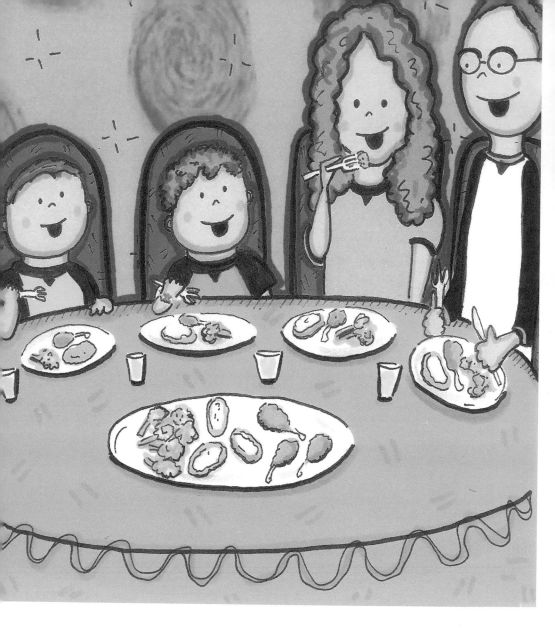

We all changed our eating habits at home to make
sure I was eating and drinking things that were
healthy for me. The nurse at the hospital also gave
me a special bracelet to wear all the time to let people
know that I am diabetic.

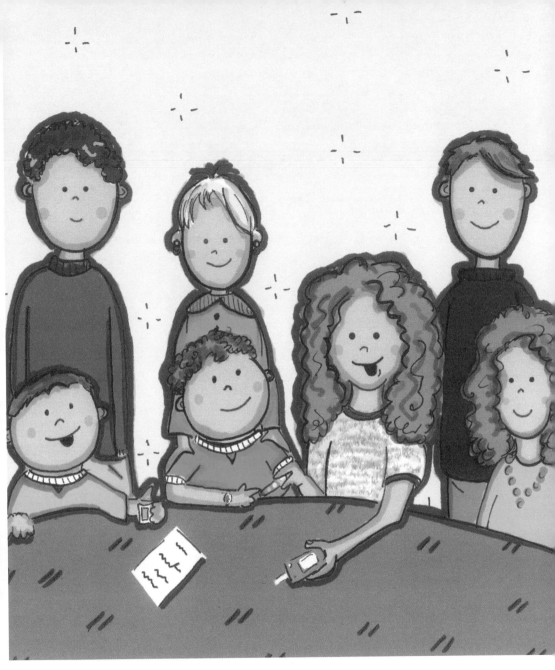

Even my aunts, uncles and grandparents learned how to test my blood before I ate, and knew that I had to have a shot after. My brother David always reminded me if I forgot.

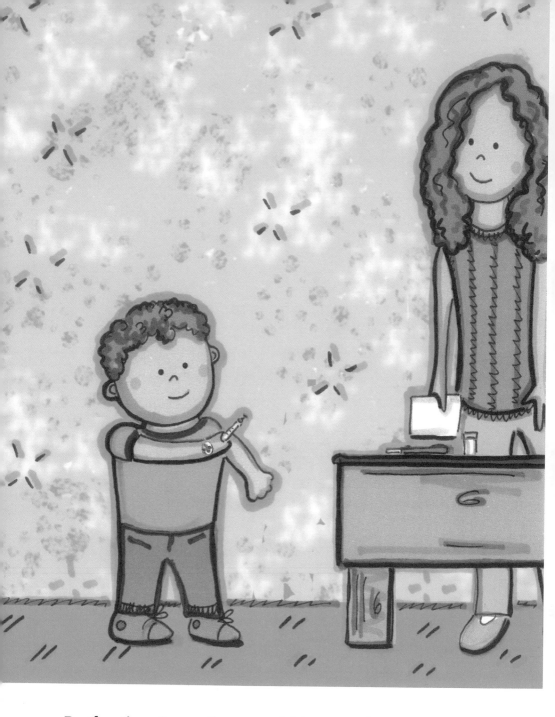

By the time I was 3 years old I was poking my own finger to test my blood, and when I turned 4 I was giving myself my own shot!

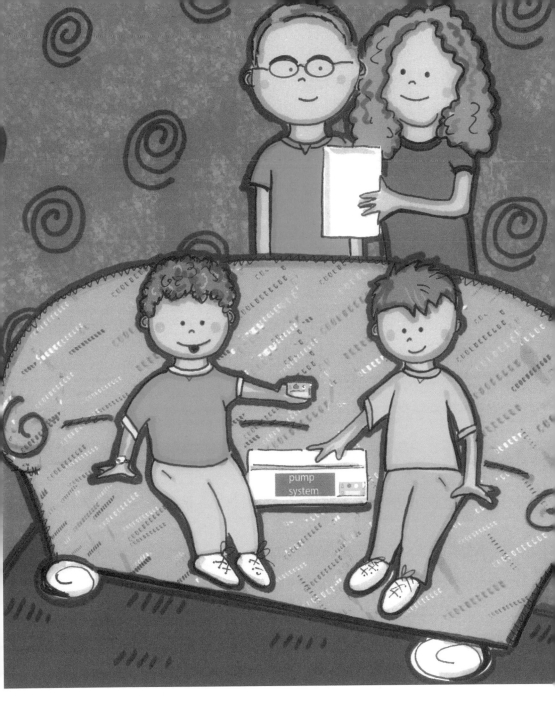

When I turned 6 my parents decided that I was old enough
to have an Insulin Pump. I was so excited because this
meant I wouldn't need shots anymore!

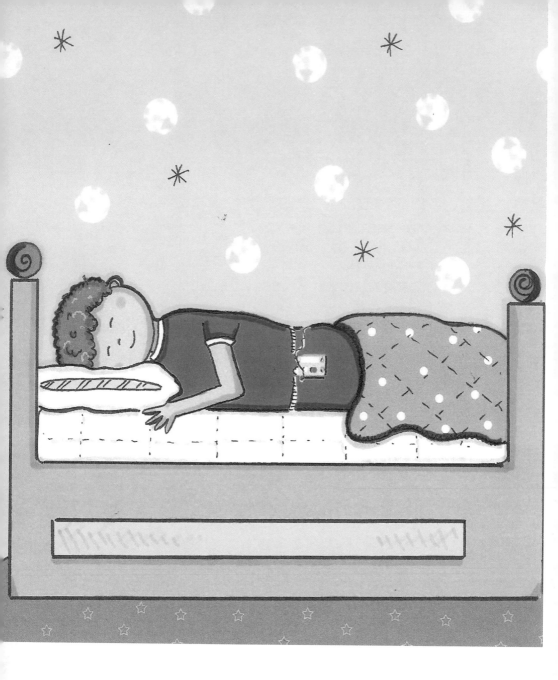

The insulin pump is attached to your body with a little tube that gives you insulin throughout the day and night. The doctors figured out what formula to use for me to make sure I was getting the right amount of insulin.

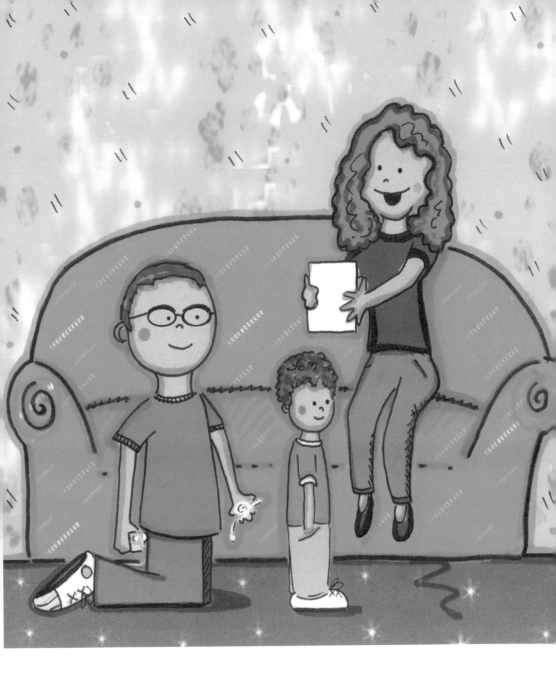

Mom and dad change the tubing on my pump every
3 days. I have my pump on all the time except when
I go swimming or take a shower.

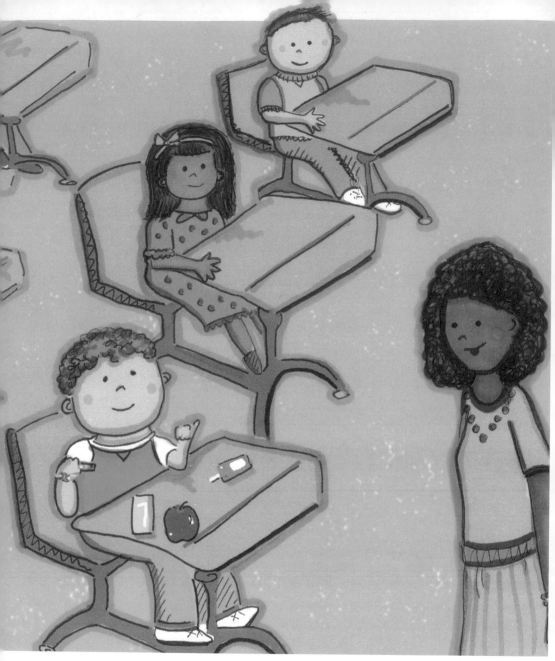

My teachers at school know all about my diabetes and how
to help take care of me. The nurse used to give me shots
when I needed them, and all my teachers know when I
need to test my blood. I bring my own healthy snacks and
lunches to school, and I keep juice boxes there just in case
my blood sugar is low.

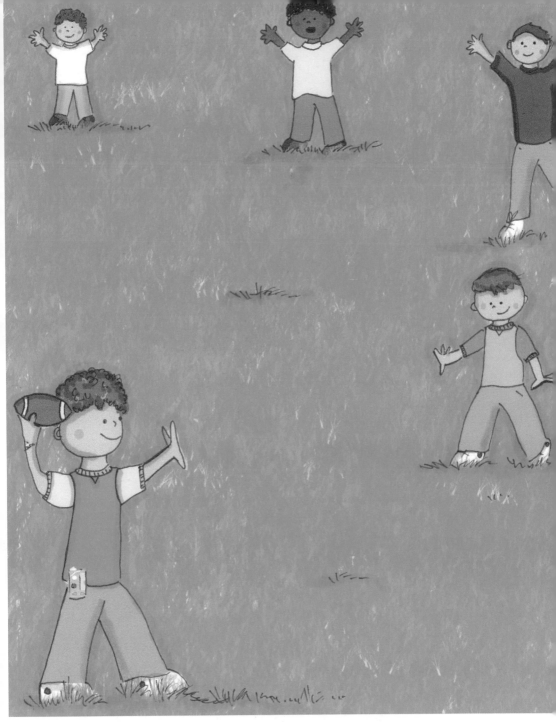

Having Type 1 Diabetes has never stopped me from doing anything I've wanted to do. I love sports and play all of them. My favorite sport is football, but I also like basketball, soccer, baseball and hockey.

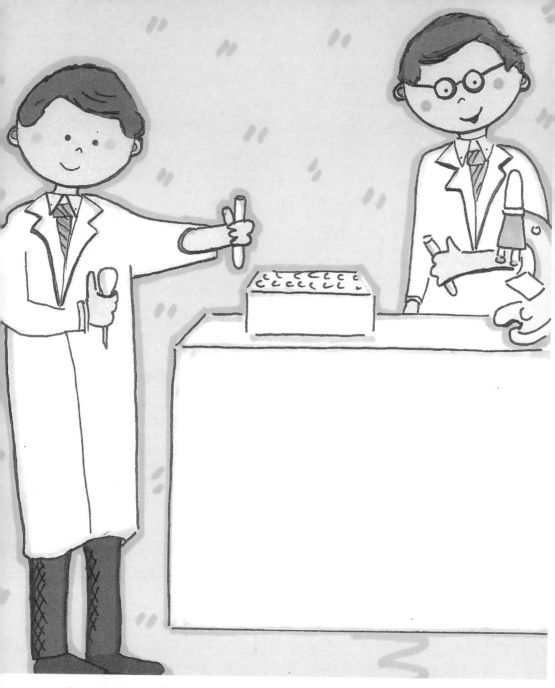

Doctors and scientists are not quite sure why some
people get Type 1 Diabetes but they are working
very hard to find a cure for it. They have found that
people with diabetes who take care of themselves
can live a long, healthy life.

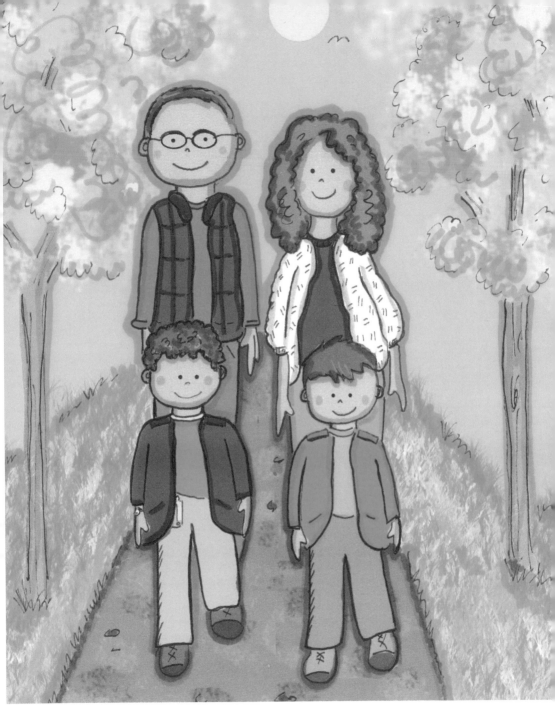

So my mom, dad and David, along with my doctors,
help to make sure I am eating right and getting lots
of exercise so we can all be a healthy family for a
long, long time.

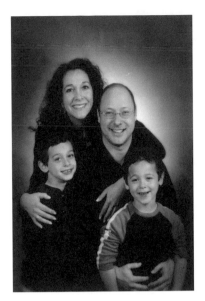

About the Author

Deanna Kleiman is the author of the children's book, "My Twin Brother".
She lives in a suburb of Detroit, Michigan, with her family.

Every year Deanna and her family and friends join thousands of people
in the Juvenile Diabetes Research Foundation Walk to help find a cure
for Juvenile Diabetes.

14654994R00018

Made in the USA
San Bernardino, CA
01 September 2014